Paulo Autran Leite Lima
Isabela Almeida Rocha
Carlos Jose O. de Matos

Evaluation of blood gases in the postoperative period of abdominal trauma

Paulo Autran Leite Lima
Isabela Almeida Rocha
Carlos Jose O. de Matos

Evaluation of blood gases in the postoperative period of abdominal trauma

The influence of heart rate

ScienciaScripts

Imprint
Any brand names and product names mentioned in this book are subject to trademark, brand or patent protection and are trademarks or registered trademarks of their respective holders. The use of brand names, product names, common names, trade names, product descriptions etc. even without a particular marking in this work is in no way to be construed to mean that such names may be regarded as unrestricted in respect of trademark and brand protection legislation and could thus be used by anyone.

Cover image: www.ingimage.com

This book is a translation from the original published under ISBN 978-613-9-61508-7.

Publisher:
Sciencia Scripts
is a trademark of
Dodo Books Indian Ocean Ltd. and OmniScriptum S.R.L publishing group

120 High Road, East Finchley, London, N2 9ED, United Kingdom
Str. Armeneasca 28/1, office 1, Chisinau MD-2012, Republic of Moldova, Europe
Printed at: see last page
ISBN: 978-620-7-63171-1

Copyright © Paulo Autran Leite Lima, Isabela Almeida Rocha, Carlos Jose O. de Matos
Copyright © 2024 Dodo Books Indian Ocean Ltd. and OmniScriptum S.R.L publishing group

Table of contents:

Chapter 1   4

Chapter 2   6

Chapter 3   12

Chapter 4   21

Chapter 5   21

Chapter 6   25

Chapter 7   32

EVALUATION OF BLOOD GASES IN THE POSTOPERATIVE PERIOD OF ABDOMINAL TRAUMA: THE INFLUENCE OF HEART RATE

Authors

PAULO AUTRAN LEITE LIMA ISABELA DE ALMEIDA ROCHA
CARLOS JOSÉ OLIVEIRA DE MATOS

Chapter 1

1 INTRODUCTION

[a]Injuries due to trauma represent the 4th leading cause of death in Brazil, with the young economically active population being the most affected. In a retrospective study carried out in the city of Aracaju from January 1998 to December 2000, it was found that of the 313 exploratory laparotomies, 61% were due to abdominal trauma, with gastric, enteric and transverse colon injuries being the most frequent.

Exploratory laparotomy is harmful because it is an invasive procedure that requires general anesthesia for the surgical procedure, corroborating the appearance of postoperative complications compared to less invasive surgical procedures such as laparoscopy.

Abdominal and laparotomic surgical procedures are very common. In the post-operative period, pulmonary complications are very common, and can reach 30 to 80%. The pathophysiological changes in the respiratory system associated with the anesthetic procedure are: a reduction in lung volume and capacity, a change in the ventilatory pattern, a change in the ventilation/perfusion ratio (V/Q), an increase in the pulmonary shunt, inefficiency in defense mechanisms such as coughing, and depression of the immune system.

Several factors should be taken into account when trying to identify patients who are potentially at risk of developing these complications, such as age, nutritional status by assessing body mass index (BMI), pre-existing respiratory diseases, smoking, duration of surgery, general anesthesia and spirometric values. Reflex inhibition of the phrenic nerve with consequent diaphragmatic paresis during the surgical procedure, causing elevation of the diaphragm and collapse of the lower lobe due to manipulation of the abdominal viscera, is perhaps the best explanation for the changes in lung volumes and capacities with repercussions on pulmonary ventilation. Arterial hypoxemia is relatively common in the postoperative period of upper abdominal surgery, which may be secondary to the duration of anesthesia and prolonged supine position on the operating table.

Post-operative pain is one of the major predisposing factors for post-operative complications, directly interfering with the ventilatory mechanics of the individual undergoing the surgical procedure. The generation of a monotonous breathing pattern directly affects the increase in lung volumes and capacities and hinders ciliary clearance, making postoperative pulmonary complications the most frequent.

General anesthesia in which patients undergo abdominal surgery has been cited as an important risk factor for respiratory changes in the postoperative period. This may be related to the presence of bronchospasm, due to endotracheal tubes directly irritating the airways, reduced thoracic expansibility, decreased lung compliance, early closure of the airways and redistribution of ventilation to the upper lung zones, which often leads to atelectasis and postoperative hypoxemia.

Changes in the behavior of arterial gases such as arterial oxygen pressure (PaO_2) and carbon dioxide pressure ($PaCO_2$) are observed in the peri- and post-operative periods, both in oxygenation and pulmonary ventilation as a result of changes in respiratory mechanics, which can be further aggravated depending on pre-established risk factors.

Arterial blood gas analysis is a tool for assessing the lung's ability to carry out gas exchange. The changes in PaO_2 and $PaCO_2$ seen in patients at rest and breathing ambient air reflect the degree to which alveolar ventilation and alveolar-capillary exchange are involved. The inverse linear relationship between the behavior of PaO_2 and $PaCO_2$ allows us to easily assess whether a given degree of arterial hypoxemia may correspond to the degree of alveolar ventilation.

Given that there is little data in the literature and in our region on the relationship between respiratory rate and arterial blood gases in the immediate post-operative period of emergency abdominal surgery caused by trauma, a period of greater attention, it is necessary to carry out research to evaluate the influence of pulmonary oxygenation and ventilation in specific situations such as exploratory laparotomy, which is important from the initial care, the surgical procedure and the follow-up and recovery period.

Chapter 2

2 ARTERIAL BLOOD GASES

Oxygen (O_2) and carbon dioxide (CO_2) are transported in the blood in different ways. Oxygen is immediately bound to hemoglobin and released into the tissues under conditions of low oxygen tension or acidosis. Very little oxygen is transported as a solution in the blood under normal pressure conditions, although this can be increased by the hyperbaric chamber. In contrast, carbon dioxide is transported in the blood entirely in solution, mostly as bicarbonate.

On average, the cell's need for oxygen is almost modest. To function effectively, a mitochondrion may need an oxygen pressure (PO_2) as low as 7.5mmHg (1Kpa). At sea level, atmospheric PO2 is 150mmHg (20Kpa) with an inspired oxygen fraction (FiO_2) equal to 0.21 and in the process of distributing oxygen to the cell there is a loss along this gradient. The first stage is the dilution of the inspired air with the expired air inside the alveolus. For each tidal volume (VT) there is a portion of gas that remains in the airways and does not come into contact with the alveolus. This is known as dead space ventilation and must be achieved before effective alveolar ventilation can occur.

The alveolar gas therefore contains a mixture of fresh gas and some expired CO_2 and the alveolar PO2 is reduced to approximately 120mmHg (16Kpa) before gas exchange begins. At the alveolar level, gas exchange involves the transfer, through the alveolar-capillary membrane, of oxygen molecules to the blood in exchange for carbon dioxide. This is accomplished by simple diffusion, which is increased in the case of oxygen due to its affinity with hemoglobin. It normally takes around 300 milliseconds (ms) for the venous blood mixture to cross a capillary and complete equilibrium often occurs in around 100 ms.

The lungs contain millions of alveolar-capillary units and adequate oxygenation depends on the coordinated and satisfactory function of the unit as a whole. The pulmonary causes of arterial hypoxemia have four main origins: hypoventilation, interference with pulmonary diffusion, uneven ventilation/peroxia and true shunt.

Hypoventilation is relatively easy to recognize due to a decrease in arterial PO2 associated with an increase in arterial PCO2. It can occur in ventilatory insufficiency associated with airway obstruction, chest wall disease and drug intoxication. Hypoxia is more related to increased pulmonary capillary transit than to diffusion failure, contributing to ventilation/perfusion (V/Q) inequality.

Hyperventilation is a physiological response to an abnormally increased respiratory drive that can be caused by a wide variety of organic, psychiatric and physiological dysfunctions or a combination of them. It is the state of increased respiration in the face of metabolic requirements, resulting in a decrease in alveolar carbon dioxide pressure ($PACO_2$) and arterial partial carbon dioxide pressure ($PaCO_2$).

Hypocapnia induces vascular constriction, resulting in a decrease in blood flow and, in response to the Bohr effect, there is an inhibition of the transfer of oxygen from circulating blood hemoglobin to tissue cells. Fluctuations in PaCO2 can have an instabilizing effect on the autonomic system, resulting in sympathetic predominance.

Altered breathing patterns can cause musculoskeletal dysfunction with subsequent chest pain that can be caused by intercostal muscle tension, spasm or fatigue, costochondritis, pain in the costovertebral or costosternal joint.

Hypoxemia (PaO2 < 55mmHg under FiO2 of 0.21) is the most threatening condition to the integrity of the human organism and must be corrected immediately, with the aim of increasing hemoglobin saturation by o2 to levels above 90%. In emergency situations, o2 should be supplied to the body at a FiO2 of 1.0 (100% o2), regardless of the patient's clinical condition or underlying pathology.

Analysis of pulmonary gas exchange makes it possible to quantify both the degree to which the respiratory system is compromised in its ability to adequately carry out gas exchange and to monitor the effectiveness of therapies aimed at improving gas exchange. Pulmonary gas exchange is a dynamic process that needs to be evaluated as a function of time. The volume expired per minute is expressed as VE and corresponds to the tidal volume expired in each respiratory cycle, multiplied by the respiratory rate (RR).

Alveolar ventilation per minute (VA) can also be expressed in the same way and corresponds to the product of the ventilation in each respiratory cycle that effectively participates in gas exchange multiplied by the respiratory rate. The amount of carbon dioxide excreted by the lung per minute (VCO_2) is proportional to the product of alveolar ventilation (VA) and the partial pressure of carbon dioxide in the alveoli (PACO2), divided by a constant K with a value of 0.863. The constant K in the equation is introduced to adjust volumes expressed under different conditions.

Therefore, alveolar ventilation is the determining factor in the levels of partial pressure of carbon dioxide in the alveolar air. Since, in practice, the partial pressure of carbon dioxide in the alveoli (PACO2) is identical to the partial pressure of carbon dioxide in the arterial blood (PaCO2), you can substitute one for the other and the balance will now be between arterial PCO2 and alveolar ventilation.

As alveolar ventilation cannot be measured directly, it can be inferred from the levels of partial pressure of carbon dioxide in arterial blood. When alveolar ventilation increases, PaCO2 decreases, and when VA decreases, PaCO2 increases. Therefore, alveolar hypoventilation is expressed by co2 retention in the alveoli and the consequent increase in the partial pressure of carbon dioxide in the alveolar air and arterial blood.

Until recently, a well-ventilated patient was one with a partial pressure of co2 below 40mmHg, thus expressing alveolar hyperventilation. This type of hyperventilation has some advantages for patients with normal respiratory mechanics. This is the case with polytraumatized patients or patients in the immediate postoperative period of major surgery, among others. However, when PaCO2 is below 35mmHg, carbon dioxide can fail to stimulate the respiratory center, which would reduce any inspiratory movement by the patient.

The partial pressure of carbon dioxide is the arterial blood gas data that expresses the magnitude of alveolar ventilation. More recently, capnography measurement of the partial pressure of carbon dioxide in alveolar air by a non-invasive method (PetCO2) has been used to assess the adequacy of alveolar ventilation. Comparative studies between PaCO2 and PetCO2 show that the non-invasive measurement is approximately a few millimeters of mercury lower than that of arterial blood.

The volume of air inspired in each respiratory cycle is called tidal air volume, and is approximately 500ml in a normal adult. After entering the upper airways, the tidal air volume is divided into two physiologically very distinct spaces. The first space, made up of approximately two thirds of the tidal air volume, is in contact with the gas-blood interface of the pulmonary circulation and is called alveolar ventilation. The remaining third is retained at the end of inhalation in the upper airways, trachea, bronchi and bronchioles, and is called dead space, in reference to its functional inactivity in terms of gas exchange.

In normal human beings at rest, the respiratory system maintains the partial pressure of carbon dioxide in the alveolar air at around 40mmHg. The partial pressure of oxygen (PO_2) in alveolar air is not regulated as precisely as PCO_2 and is lower than the PO_2 of the inspired air. As diffusion depends on the oxygen partial pressure gradient between the alveolus and the capillary, the alveolar PO_2 is never lower than the pulmonary capillary PO_2.

The passage of oxygen from the alveolus to the capillaries is made by a gas partial pressure gradient. The alveolar-arterial gradient is calculated by the simple difference between the partial pressure of oxygen in the alveolus and the partial pressure of oxygen in the arterial blood. The alveolar-arterial gradient in normal individuals is not fixed throughout the oxygen concentration scale, but increases progressively with increasing FiO_2. In patients with impaired pulmonary gas exchange, the alveolar-arterial gradient will be increased throughout the FiO_2 range, and can reach much higher values than in normal individuals.

The oxygenated index (O.I.), which does not require the calculation of alveolar oxygen pressure (PAO_2), is an easier parameter to calculate. Some studies reported the use of the oxygenated ratio (PaO_2 / $\%FiO_2$). This was subsequently changed to PaO_2/FiO_2. It is currently considered adequate when above 400, abnormal when below 300 and severely compromised when below 200. Unlike the alveolar-arterial gradient and the arterio-alveolar ratio, the O.I. is affected by changes in $PaCO_2$. This index has gained popularity due to its ease of calculation at the bedside.

The measurement of respiratory rate acts as a marker of respiratory effort, and it is necessary to monitor it more intensively in critically ill patients, where most adults cannot tolerate certain rates of more than 30 strokes per minute for long, due to the inherent risk of muscle exhaustion and metabolic reserves, which is directly related to changes in lung volume.

2.1 Blood gas analysis

The difference between the two forms of metabolic gas transport is fundamental when interpreting arterial blood gas measurements. The cell requires oxygen to survive, but the transport of oxygen in the blood will have no effect on the organism if it has not been delivered. On the contrary, the chemistry involved in transporting carbon dioxide controls the body's acid-base status in the short term. When considering arterial blood gas, it is best to examine these functions separately.

The assessment of acid-base status requires measurements of arterial blood gas pressures. The gas analyzer measures the average level of PO_2, PCO_2 and pH and subsequently calculates the values of bicarbonate, standard bicarbonate and base excess using the Henderson-Hasselbach equation. The interpretation of acid-base status requires an examination of PaCO2 and pH.

Abnormalities are described in terms of their production. A respiratory acidosis resulting from hypoventilation shows a low pH and a high PaCO2. If this condition persists for some time, serum bicarbonate will become elevated and the acid will be excreted by the kidneys to compensate. In cases of nocturnal hypoventilation, the daytime PaO2 may be normal, but the elevation of the base excess provides clues to the ventilatory history. If an alkalosis (high pH) is associated with a low PaCO2, this is due to voluntary hyperventilation, respiratory alkalosis.

The development of acid products in diabetes or renal failure results in low pH and bicarbonate, along with a metabolic acidosis. Finally, the loss of acid from the stomach through prolonged vomiting can produce metabolic alkalosis, characterized by high pH and bicarbonate and normal PaCO2. These outlines of gasometric changes are superficial interpretations, but they provide a useful basis for clinical management in many circumstances.

Arterial blood gas not only provides an indication of oxygenation and carbon dioxide elimination, but also of acid-base status. Many automatic blood gas machines only measure pH, pO2 and pCO2 and extrapolate these values to bicarbonate and oxygen saturation. These extrapolations are accurate under many circumstances, but oxygen saturation can be misleading in the presence of carboxyhaemoglobin. Hypoxemia (PO2 less than 60mmHg) and hypercarbia (PaCO2 greater than 45mmHg) are easy to recognize.

In simple terms, in acidosis the pH is always low (normal pH is 7.36 - 7.44) and in alkalosis the pH is always high (remembering that pH is the inverse and is the logarithmic expression of the hydrogen ion concentration). The metabolic causes of acidosis and alkalosis involve a primary change in bicarbonate concentration and the respiratory causes involve a change in PaCO2.
Arterial blood gas provides an accurate measure of the uptake of oxygen and elimination of carbon dioxide by the respiratory system as a whole. Arterial blood is often taken from the radial artery at the wrist. Rarely, arterialized capillary samples can be taken from the ear lobe. Blood gas is best used as a measure of gas exchange in the baseline state, so it is imperative that the patient rests, calmly, with an inspired oxygen level (FiO2) prior to collection. Normal blood gas values are: pH- 7.35 - 7.45; PaO2: 80 - 100 mmHg (10.7 - 13.3KPa); PaCO2: 35 - 45mmHg (4.7 - 6.0KPa); HCO_3^- : 22 - 26mmol/l; Base excess: -2 - +2.

Blood samples to assess gas exchange parameters have been used for over 30 years. Depending on the need, these samples can be obtained from blood gas by percutaneous puncture of a peripheral artery, with a permanent catheter (arterial, central venous or pulmonary artery) or by capillary sampling.

The results obtained from arterial blood gas analysis are essential for the diagnosis and treatment of oxygen and acid-base disorders. Arterial blood gas analysis is considered the gold standard of gas exchange analysis, against which all other methods are compared.

The main parameters of pH, PCO2 and PO2 in a blood sample are measured with a blood gas analyzer. Analyzers use these measurements to calculate various secondary values, such as plasma bicarbonate, base excess or deficit and hemoglobin saturation.

2.2 Acid-base disorder

2.2.1 Respiratory Acidosis

It is defined as any physiological process that increases arterial PCO2 (>45mmHg) and decreases arterial pH (<7.35). Increased PaCO2 (hypercapnia) decreases arterial pH because dissolved CO_2 produces carbonic acid.

$$CO_2 + H_2O \rightarrow H_2CO_3 \rightarrow HCO_3^- + H^+$$

Any process in which alveolar ventilation cannot eliminate co2 at the same rate as the body produces it causes respiratory acidosis. If hypercapnia is decompensated, acidosis occurs with a low pH, a high PaCO2 and a normal or slightly elevated [HCO3-]. Renal compensation for respiratory acidosis begins as soon as the PaCO2 level rises. The kidneys absorb HCO3- from the renal tubular filtrate, bringing the arterial pH into the normal range; this process can take several days.

2.2.2 Respiratory alkalosis

It occurs when a physiological process lowers arterial PCO2 (< 35 mmHg). A low PaCO2 (hypocapnia) forces the hydration reaction to the left, decreasing the concentration of carbonic acid and increasing the pH:

$$CO_2 + H_2O \leftarrow H_2CO_3 \leftarrow HCO_3^- + H^+$$

This process occurs when the ventilatory elimination of co2 exceeds its production. Possible causes of hyperventilation are anxiety, fever, stimulant drugs, pain and central nervous system damage. The kidneys compensate for respiratory alkalosis by excreting HCO3- in the urine, and complete compensation can take days. When partially compensated, it is characterized by a low PaCO2, a low [HCO3-] and an alkaline pH.

2.2.3 Metabolic Acidosis

It can be defined as any process that lowers plasma [HCO3-]. Reducing [HCO3-] lowers blood pH because it reduces the amount of bases in relation to the amount of acids in the blood. There are two ways of producing a metabolic acidosis: - accumulation of fixed acids in the blood, in conditions of low blood flow in which tissue hypoxia and anaerobic metabolism produce lactic acid; - excessive loss of HCO3- from the

diarrhea is a typical example. Hyperventilation is the main compensatory mechanism for metabolic acidosis.

2.2.4 Metabolic alkalosis

This can be characterized by an increase in plasma [HCO3-], loss of H ions+ and an elevated pH. An elevated [HCO3-] is not always diagnostic of metabolic alkalosis because it can be due to renal compensation for respiratory acidosis. The most frequent causes may be loss of fixed acids or gain of base cap in the blood.

The expected compensatory response to metabolic alkalosis is hypoventilation (CO_2 retention). Metabolic alkalosis apparently attenuates the hypoxemic stimulus to ventilation. However, individuals with low PaO2 levels (up to 50mmHg) can hypoventilate at high PaCO2 levels (up to 60mmHg) to compensate for alkalosis.

Chapter 3

3 LAPAROTOMIES

Surgery can be considered the oldest branch of therapy. It possibly began in prehistoric times, with primitive man when, in the struggle for survival, he suffered some kind of injury and, consequently, some kind of treatment. Thus, laparotomy was defined as the surgical opening of the peritoneal cavity or as a surgical maneuver involving an incision through the abdominal wall to access the abdominal cavity.

The ease with which the surgeon can act in the operative field when performing abdominal surgery is directly related to the access route chosen. Poor exposure, making the operation uncomfortable or hindering necessary maneuvers, can lead to problems at the end of the operation which will have a negative impact on the final result.

The indication for laparotomy can be described in the following circumstances: to treat an already diagnosed intra-abdominal lesion; to treat an unknown intra-abdominal lesion (exploratory laparotomy); as an auxiliary means, in the treatment of another extra-abdominal lesion (for example, gastrotomies for oesophageal stenosis) and to drain the cavity.

The general and fundamental principles of good surgical technique have not changed. Thus, asepsis, hemostasis, preservation of circulation, delicacy, tension-free sutures and obliteration of dead spaces are indispensable factors in a correct laparotomy. The ideal incision should provide satisfactory access to the affected organ via the chosen route, be of adequate size, allowing work to be done without dragging on the viscera according to the patient's biotype and the injury to be treated; be made with perfect hemostasis, avoiding the formation of hematomas which would hinder healing and which could lead to dehiscence of the wall; avoid severing nerves in the wall; facilitate closure without compromising the solidity of the wall; facilitate good drainage; leave as aesthetic a scar as possible.

The types of incisions can be made according to the location. The median incision consists of opening the wall in the midline, through the Alba line, and can be superior (xipho-umbilical or supra-umbilical), inferior (from the umbilical scar to the pubis or infra-umbilical) or extensive (xipho-pubic).

The median supra-umbilical incision is the oldest type of abdominal incision. Visualization of the organs of the upper abdomen (gallbladder, stomach, hepatic hilum, pancreas, duodenum) is perfect and there is a possibility of easy enlargement, but there is a risk of easy formation of an incisional hernia due to the posterior traction of the lateral abdominal muscles.

The infra-umbilical median incision is most commonly used in gynecological laparotomies. Access to the pelvic organs and appendages (intestinal loops, Muller's ducts, pelvic cavity, aorta) is excellent. The main precaution is to properly remove the bladder, which is in the lower angle of the incision, masked by the pre-vesical fat.

The paramedian type consists of penetrating the cavity by opening the sheaths of the rectus abdominis muscle. It can be transmuscular, with longitudinal section of the rectus abdominis muscle or internal or external pararectal. It can also be divided into a supra-umbilical paramedian pararectal incision to approach the organs of the upper abdomen (gallbladder, hepatic hilum, stomach, barium), which can be made either to the right or left of the midline. It has advantages in terms of visualization and the possibility of widening, which makes it more difficult for an incisional hernia to form.

The infra-umbilical paramedian pararectal incision can also be made to the right or left of the infra-umbilical midline, starting at the level of the umbilical scar, about 3 cm from the outer edge of the anterior rectus muscle, and proceeding parallel downwards. This is the ideal incision for cases of acute abdomen, such as appendicitis.

Another classification is the combined type, which consists of associating two or more of the incisions mentioned above, with the aim of enlarging the operative region. The use of incisions of this type is less frequent and depends on the surgeon's experience when exploring the cavity. After selecting the type of incision, the abdominal wall is opened, strictly following the systematization of the procedure, where any access adopted must be of adequate size, without hesitating to enlarge the incision if necessary.

After opening the abdominal cavity, the contents are rigorously examined and explored manually, examining from quadrant to quadrant, trying to identify lesions of greater or lesser importance, deciding whether or not there is a need to increase the incision already made in the wall or to make a combined incision for better exposure. The organ or tumour is then exteriorized, if possible, by appropriate mobilization, ending with surgical treatment of the lesion that prompted the intervention.

As an invasive method of treatment, surgery can present risks that prolong the patient's recovery. As a result, some complications can arise from laparotomies. Bleeding, due to poor technique and lack of attention when ligating vessels, requires immediate intervention to locate and correct. Other complications such as epithelialization deficiency, which is prone to infection, and hypoproteinemia, can be the cause of wall dehiscence, in addition to the painful condition, which will lead to complications in other systems.

3.1 Anesthetics in Abdominal Surgery

The anesthetic procedure can be regional or general, but the anesthetic technique of choice for upper abdominal surgery is general anesthesia, which can be defined as a state in which certain physiological systems of the body are subjected to external regulatory conditions, by the action of various chemical agents associated with tracheal intubation and controlled ventilation to ensure protection of the airway and adequate pulmonary ventilation (normocarbia).

In the pre-anesthetic assessment of patients undergoing abdominal surgery, in addition to the usual items, such as past history, research into previous concomitant pathologies, allergies, medications used by the patient and addictions (smoking, alcoholism, toxic substances), it is necessary to observe particular situations, which are related to the most frequent causes of these surgeries.

In abdominal surgery, the patient should be monitored according to the extent of the procedure, the severity of the clinical situation, as well as the possibility of abrupt changes in blood volume, changes in pulmonary ventilation and hydroelectrolytic balance. Special attention should be paid to: body temperature, due to the extent of the exposed surgical area, which favors heat loss; neuromuscular transmission, due to the need for muscle relaxation; blood gas levels (especially carbon dioxide - CO_2) in laparoscopic surgeries.

Cardiac monitoring should be used in all patients. The handling of viscera and the peritoneal cavity causes changes in the intensity of the surgical stimulus, with the appearance of reflex responses from the autonomic nervous system. Measuring direct arterial pressure is essential for hemodynamic control in critically ill patients and in cases where major bleeding is expected. In surgeries where there are rapid changes in blood volume and hydroelectrolytic balance, the measurement of central venous pressure is essential in critically ill patients. This indication in abdominal surgery is related to the patient's cardiovascular conditions, as well as the compartmental changes that may occur.

Pulse oximetry is now part of the routine monitoring of all anesthetic procedures, especially major abdominal surgeries. Its indication extends to the recovery room or ICU (Intensive Care Center) in the post-operative period. Capnometry is mandatory monitoring in laparoscopic abdominal surgery. It is through capnometry that an early diagnosis of hypercarbia can be made.

Recovery from anesthesia according to appropriate criteria, such as awakening and restoration of protective airway reflexes as soon as the surgery is over, is the desired goal in most cases of abdominal surgery. To this end, inhalation anesthetics should be discontinued 10-30 minutes before the end of surgery, depending on the agent used. Factors such as solubility, anesthetic uptake, cardiac output, ventilation, temperature, oxygen intake flow and diffusion hypoxia influence the time required for recovery from anesthesia.

3.2 Systemic Repercussions of Anesthesia

Anesthesia is a procedure with a potential risk of serious complications, respiratory complications being the main cause of morbidity and mortality. Basically, 75% of these complications are due to ventilation failure and difficulty or failure in tracheal intubation. Hypoxemia and hypercapnia are the most important consequences of these adverse situations.

The mechanisms for producing hypoxemia can be divided into two groups according to the level of alveolar oxygen pressure (PaO_2): with decreased alveolar oxygen pressure and without decreased alveolar oxygen pressure. PaO_2 will decrease in proportion to the reduction in alveolar oxygen pressure (PAO_2) caused by a decrease in FiO_2 or a reduction in alveolar ventilation (hypoventilation). A decrease in FiO_2 is usually associated with mechanical failures in the oxygen supply, such as cylinders, valves, pressure gauges, flow meters, etc.

Hypoventilation is the most common cause of hypoxemia in the post-anesthetic period. In the transoperative period, if the patient is on spontaneous ventilation, anesthetic depression is the main cause of hypoventilation; in controlled ventilation, the most common causes are equipment failures (malfunctioning fans, valves, disconnections, among others).

The induction of anesthesia causes an alteration in the V/Q ratio which is manifested by an increase in the alveolar-arterial oxygen difference ($P_{(A-a)}O_2$), mainly due to the action of inhaled anesthetics which block the vasoconstrictor response of the pulmonary circulation to hypoxia, causing a decrease in P_{aO_2}. A FiO2 of at least 0.3 is recommended in order to prevent hypoxemia during general anesthesia.

The increase in the alveolar-arterial oxygen difference is also associated with the reduction in functional residual capacity (FRC) that occurs at the start of anesthesia. FRC is reduced by changing the patient's position and is more pronounced in elderly, obese, pregnant, pneumopathic and congenital heart disease patients.

Surgical anesthesia is closely related to the hypoxemia that occurs in the postoperative period. The magnitude and duration of hypoxemia will depend on the site and duration of the surgery. A significant drop in PaO2 can occur in thoracic and upper abdominal surgeries. Obesity, advanced age, pain, abdominal distension, hypothermia and pneumopathies are predisposing factors for hypoxemia in the postoperative period.

In the immediate post-operative period, the administration of humidified oxygen to all patients via face masks or nasal catheters is recommended. The use of a pulse oximeter is of fundamental importance both during and after anesthesia, and since 1994 the American Society of Anesthesiologists has made this monitoring mandatory in recovery rooms.

Hypercapnia is another consequence of the anesthetic effect in the postoperative period and its causes include: a) increased endogenous production of CO_2 caused by fever, sepsis, malignant hyperthermia, convulsive crisis and excessive production of catecholamines; b) exogenous administration of CO_2 in laparoscopic procedures when alveolar ventilation is not adequate; c) an increase in the inspired CO_2 fraction and an increase in respiratory dead space, such as failures in the anesthesia machine; d) a decrease in alveolar ventilation, whether caused centrally, peripherally or related to airway obstruction and lung diseases.

Some degree of hypoventilation is common during recovery from anesthesia. Central respiratory depression is the main cause of increased P_{aCO_2}. In the immediate postoperative period, hypoventilation can be caused mainly by overdose of anesthetics, exaggerated hyperventilation during anesthesia and hypothermia. Although moderate hypercapnia is well tolerated in healthy patients, increases in PaCO2 are dangerous and can cause respiratory acidosis, arrhythmias and altered level of consciousness.

There are no specific clinical signs of hypercapnia. In the awake patient, breathing spontaneously, a PaCO2 of 50mmHg will produce a cardiovascular response that translates into increased inotropism, heart rate, stroke volume and decreased peripheral vascular resistance. General anesthesia and high spinal blockade reduce the intensity of this response. Diagnosis of hypercapnia is confirmed by arterial blood gas with PaCO2 measurement and by capnometry and capnography, which allow continuous control of end-expired CO_2.

During anesthesia and surgery, the cardiovascular system is subjected to multiple aggressions resulting from the direct or indirect effect of anesthetic agents, changes in respiration, temperature, blood volume and the activity of the autonomic nervous system. These alterations are well tolerated by an intact cardiovascular system, but patients with cardiovascular disease can suffer from manifest decompensation, such as myocardial ischemia, pulmonary congestion and arrhythmias.

Acute renal failure (ARF) is an important cause of post-operative morbidity and mortality, especially in major surgery. Its incidence ranges from 0.1 to 30% and mortality exceeds 50%. In the perioperative period, almost half of patients can develop ARF, requiring acute dialysis.

Different anesthetic-surgical factors contribute to the decrease in urinary volume in the transoperative period: a) the effect of anesthetic-surgical stress with increased catecholamines that reduce renal blood flow (RBF) and increased secretion of antidiuretic hormone (ADH); b) surgical compression of vessels or aortic clamping, including infrarenal; c) hypothermia; d) reduced cardiac output and RBF promoted by mechanical ventilation; e) direct or indirect effects of anesthetic drugs. Anesthetic drugs that depress the myocardium and cause vasodilation reduce blood pressure and will indirectly reduce FSR. Hemodynamic changes and urine output are used to monitor renal function transoperatively, but are not ideal because they are indirect measures.

Central nervous system (CNS) complications that occur after anesthesia can be divided into: a) those dependent on anesthesia and the clinical characteristics of the patients (delayed recovery of consciousness, post-operative delirium, seizures and strokes); b) those associated with specific surgical procedures (carotid endarterectomies, cardiac and aortic surgeries).

Prolonged action of anesthetic drugs, metabolic abnormalities and neurological damage are the main situations associated with delayed recovery of consciousness after anesthesia. Factors such as advanced age, obesity, liver and kidney failure, hypothermia, hypothyroidism and drug interactions are associated with prolonged action of anesthetics. The use of alcohol and illicit drugs is also associated with moderate awakening.

A neurological examination can be carried out in the recovery room in order to rule out more serious causes. Little information can be obtained in these circumstances, and it only serves as a preliminary assessment. Even neurologically normal patients show abnormal eye reflexes and movements when they wake up from anesthesia. The presence of unilateral abnormal reflexes draws attention to a possible neurological injury. The delay in waking up caused by drugs, although undesirable, does not pose any major risks to the patient, as long as adequate ventilation and circulatory parameters are maintained.

The presence of neurological damage or metabolic abnormalities is suspected if unconsciousness persists after a reasonable waiting time or if there is no response to the diagnostic test with antagonists. The patient's previous history may raise the suspicion of an unrecognized neurological lesion. A history of cerebral ischemia, seizure disorders and drug use should be investigated.

3.3 The post-operative period in abdominal surgery

Care must be taken when extubating patients undergoing emergency abdominal surgery. Many of these patients undergo surgery after a poor preoperative assessment. It is therefore preferable for the cannula to be removed in the post-anesthetic recovery unit or intensive care unit. An arterial blood gas measurement may be useful before the tube is removed.

Vital data should be monitored every 15 minutes until completely stabilized.

Thereafter, the intervals are spread out. In the first few hours after the operation, the horizontal dorsal decubitus position, without a pillow, is the most recommended. Once conscious, the patient is encouraged to change position at short intervals. Active movement of the limbs is imperative until the patient is able to walk.

Oral food intake is maintained in the immediate postoperative period. The reintroduction of an oral liquid diet depends on the type of surgery performed. Cholecystectomies and appendectomies (without perforation of the cecal appendix) generally do not prevent an early start. In cases of proximal digestive anastomoses or gas distension of the intestine, the diet is reintroduced after the reappearance of hydroaerial noises and anal elimination of flatus. The reintroduction of the diet should be progressive, moving successively from liquid to pasty and finally solid foods.

The use of the nasogastric catheter has been declining over time and its indications are limited to elective procedures. It is an effective instrument for draining secretions and gases, decompressing the digestive tract, but its incorrect attachment damages the wing of the nose and prolonged use predisposes to the development of reflux oesophagitis, and it should be removed as soon as possible.

In the post-operative period, once the anesthetic agents have worn off, the patient experiences pain. In operations on the body's natural cavities, this pain is due to skin damage to deep parietal structures and viscera. The intensity of the symptom depends on the physiological and psychological characteristics of the patient and their tolerance to pain, the site and nature of the operation and the intensity of the surgical trauma.

In emergency operations, it is not always possible to explain post-operative events in detail. The site and nature of the operation are also relevant. Surgical procedures on the upper abdomen and chest are usually accompanied by more severe pain. The type of incision should also be taken into account, as incisions that involve severing several nerves are accompanied by more internal pain in the post-operative period. Pain inhibits post-operative movement and excessive sedation depresses breathing.

Wound infections occur in approximately % of cases in infected surgeries. In acute abdominal trauma, the rate of wound infection is high, even in the absence of contamination. Trauma victims have other aggravating factors, such as tissue hypoxia due to hypovolemia, loss of defense elements against infection, such as fibronectin, during hemorrhage.

Surgical wound dehiscence occurs in around 3% of cases, so the type of incision seems to play an important role. This is why dehiscence is common in longitudinal laparotomies and uncommon in transverse abdominal incisions. Other factors, such as abdominal distension and coughing, also contribute to dehiscence and evisceration. Most eviscerations occur between the 4th and 10th postoperative day. The elimination of a serosanguinous exudate is the main clinical sign and treatment consists of resuturing with "mass" stitches.

Post-operative complications are defined as a second unexpected illness that occurs up to thirty days after surgery, altering the patient's clinical condition and making therapeutic intervention necessary, whether or not with medication. It also includes the exacerbation of pre-existing illnesses whose accentuation of symptoms constitutes a type of post-operative complication.

Although pulmonary and cardiac complications are more frequent, other types of complications can occur, such as wall infection, urinary infection, thromboembolic complications, renal failure, stroke, bleeding disorders and decompensation of endocrinopathies.

In most studies that have used well-defined and reliable scientific methodology, the following are considered to be pulmonary complications: acute respiratory infection, including pneumonia and tracheobronchitis; atelectasis; acute respiratory failure; bronchospasm; orotracheal intubation and mechanical ventilation for more than 48 hours.

Studies carried out in the 1970s and 1980s showed that atelectasis was the most frequent post-operative complication and its incidence ranged from 7% to 35%. Respiratory infections have been the most frequent post-operative pulmonary complications, with pneumonia leading this incidence and also being the main cause of post-operative mortality, in agreement with the majority of authors.

Pulmonary complications are the result of changes in lung function that occur in the postoperative period of abdominal and thoracic surgery. They can be grouped into four categories: changes in lung volume and capacity, ventilatory pattern, gas exchange and pulmonary defenses. In the first 24 to 48 hours after surgery with an operative incision above the umbilical scar, there is a decrease in vital capacity (VC) of up to 60% of its preoperative value and a progressive return to its pre-surgical level within one to two weeks.

Ventilatory dysfunction is independent of the extent or type of surgical incision, since in upper abdominal surgeries using laparoscopy there is also a decrease of up to 36% in VC on the first day after the surgical procedure. What differentiates surgery with a conventional incision from laparoscopy is the earlier return of ventilatory function, which occurs between the third and sixth day in the latter surgical modality.

In abdominal surgery with a laparotomy incision, there is a decrease in tidal volume of up to 25% of its preoperative value, associated with an increase of up to 20% in respiratory rate, while maintaining the minute volume unchanged, and this is more frequent in the first 24 hours after surgery.

The arterial hypoxemia observed in the postoperative period is aggravated by secretion retention and narrowing of the airways, leading to the closure of dependent pulmonary zones and the predominance of areas with a low ventilation-perfusion ratio. For this reason, arterial blood oxygen pressure (PaO_2) can decrease by approximately 30% compared to its pre-operative value.

Acute carbon dioxide (CO_2) retention is a problem seen more frequently in patients with COPD (chronic obstructive pulmonary disease), whose lung reserve is limited, or who already have chronic hypercapnia. Hypocapnia usually occurs due to a change in the ventilatory pattern. The decrease in mucociliary clearance seen in the postoperative period is due to cough inhibition, prolonged immobilization, orotracheal intubation and the action of drugs such as narcotics.

Patients with respiratory symptoms such as coughing, expectoration and wheezing have a higher incidence of post-operative pulmonary complications. In studies, symptomatic patients had 2.9 times more pulmonary complications than non-symptomatic patients. According to several authors, pneumopathies increase the risk of pulmonary morbidity and mortality in any surgical procedure.

The length of surgery is one of the main risk factors that should be checked during the preoperative assessment. It was observed that surgical procedures lasting more than five hours were associated with an increased risk of developing heart failure and death from non-cardiac causes. In patients with a history of heart disease, there is a direct association between the length of surgery and the occurrence of cardiac complications.

Surgical procedures lasting more than three hours are associated with a higher risk of developing post-operative pulmonary complications. Intra-abdominal, non-cardiac thoracic and vascular surgical procedures are associated with increased mortality and post-operative cardiopulmonary morbidity when compared to other types of surgery. Patients undergoing extra-cardiac, abdominal, thoracic and vascular surgery have a two-fold increase in the risk of cardiac death and a six-fold increase in the risk of non-fatal post-operative cardiac complications.

Cardiac complications can also be frequent in patients undergoing abdominal surgery, with alterations in rhythm and rate being secondary to the depth of the anesthetic plane, alterations in the autonomic nervous system, the direct effect of anesthetics and mechanical stimulation resulting from intubation and tracheal disintubation. The higher incidence of heart rhythm disturbances during anesthesia seems to be related to the presence of heart disease and previous arrhythmias, advanced age, mechanical ventilation, the use of digitalis and surgeries lasting more than three hours.

Patients with previous heart disease can suffer from cardiogenic shock after upper abdominal surgery, which can lead to heart failure and acute myocardial infarction. The hypotension that occurs during surgery, caused mainly by the action of anesthetic agents and surgical stress, reduces myocardial wall tension, decreases oxygen consumption and alters blood flow to the coronary arteries. However, this reduction can exceed the self-regulatory limit, further decreasing blood flow to the coronaries, which can lead to worsening or new ischemic dysfunction.

Studies have shown pulmonary alterations in the postoperative period of upper abdominal surgery and exploratory laparotomy, respectively, demonstrating a drop in vital capacity (VC), forced expiratory volume in the first second (FEV1) by spirometry before and after surgery.

Dyspnea in the post-operative period is common, mainly due to the onset of post-operative complications, and can be related to multiple symptoms reported as a feeling of discomfort when breathing. It is difficult to measure for those assisting the patient, but can be facilitated when markers such as RR are measured.

Individuals undergoing upper abdominal surgery may experience some pulmonary repercussions caused by anesthesia and the surgical procedure itself. Both can accentuate the reduction in functional residual capacity (FRC), promoting early closure of the small airways, leading to a degree of hypoxemia and possible incidence of atelectasis, alterations in respiratory mechanics, gas exchange, breathing pattern and pulmonary defense mechanisms, leading to the appearance of postoperative pulmonary complications (PPC).

Chapter 4

4 OBJECTIVES

4.1 General

- To analyze the influence of respiratory rate on arterial blood gases in the immediate postoperative period of exploratory laparotomy due to abdominal trauma.

4.2 Specifics

• Observe arterial gas pressure concentrations ($PaCO_2$ and PaO_2), respiratory rate and oxygenation index in the first three days after surgery.

• To assess whether there is a correlation between respiratory rate and arterial blood gases and arterial carbon dioxide pressure and arterial oxygen pressure in the first three days after exploratory laparotomy for abdominal trauma.

Chapter 5

5 CASUISTRY AND METHODS

5.1 Sample

We evaluated adult patients (aged >18 years) of both sexes admitted to the Trauma Center of the Hospital Governador Joao Alves Filho in the city of Aracaju-SE and submitted to exploratory laparotomy for abdominal trauma.

All the patients who underwent laparotomy were admitted to the General Surgery department in the emergency department of the aforementioned hospital. After receiving the patient, he or she was submitted to a 1ª assessment according to the ATLS by the on-call doctor, and a request was made to the on-call general surgeon, who assessed the need for intervention and, when indicated, the patient was referred to the operating room.

Patients underwent surgery under general anesthesia with a balanced technique, using intravenous and inhaled drugs, combined with inducing agents and muscle relaxants (propofol or etomidate + fentanyl + pancuronium + isofluorane and nitrous oxide). After the surgery, the patient remained in the surgical recovery unit, post-anesthetic recovery service (PACU) and was referred to surgical nursing on the 1st post-operative day after stabilization of the clinical-surgical procedure. Depending on the patient's needs, intravenous analgesics could be administered in the post-operative period.

5.2 Inclusion and Exclusion Criteria

Patients were included in the study after a critical analysis of the surgical-anesthetic procedure and the type of emergency abdominal surgery performed. Criteria for inclusion in the study were: general anesthesia, anesthesia time greater than or equal to 120 minutes, emergency surgery such as exploratory laparotomy with xipho-pubic incision. The exclusion criteria were: chest surgery associated with trauma, hemodynamic alterations, previous cardiorespiratory pathologies, renal disorders presented during or after surgery in the first three postoperative days.

5.3 Ethical considerations

The study was approved by the Human Research Ethics Committee of the Federal University of Sergipe (UFS) and cleared after analysis of the project by the Continuing Education Center (CEC) of the Governador Joao Alves Filho Hospital. All the patients or responsible companions involved in the research were informed of its objectives and, if they agreed, signed the Informed Consent Form.

5.4 Research Methods

This was a field study with a non-experimental cohort design of an analytical and descriptive nature, in which data was collected between April and September 2005 during the first three days of the post-operative period.

5.5 Variables surveyed

- Age;
- Anesthesia time;
- Surgery time;
- Respiratory rate (RR);
- Arterial carbon dioxide pressure ($PaCO_2$);
- Arterial oxygen pressure (PaO_2);
- Oxygenation index (O.I.);

5.6 Data collection

All patients were initially assessed in order to analyze the criteria for inclusion in the study using an assessment/monitoring form, after which the following steps were followed:

$>$ Measurement of variables:
- All patients were on room respiration (FiO_2 at 21%).
- Respiratory rate was measured 3 to 5 minutes before arterial blood sampling.
- Arterial blood was collected preferentially from the radial artery up to three attempts. In conditions where this access was unfeasible, priority was given to puncturing the femoral artery.
- Before the arterial blood sample was taken, the patient was properly reassured about the test and instructed on the relevant procedures.
- After the arterial blood was collected, it was analyzed in less than 5 minutes, taking care to transport it and eliminate possible air bubbles and contamination.
- The same times were set for the collection of arterial blood and the other variables. The data was recorded on an individual monitoring form.

$>$ Calculation of the Oxygenation Index (O.I.):

$$IO = \frac{PaO_2}{FiO_2 \text{ (fraction of inspired oxygen)}}$$

$>$ Arterial puncture according to the American Association for Respiratory Care (AARC):
- Wash hands and wear protective barriers (gloves)
- Position the patient, extending their wrist to approximately 30°.
- Clean the area thoroughly with 70% isopropyl alcohol
- Heparinize the syringe and remove the excess (anticoagulant: heparin lithium or heparin sodium).
- Palpate and hold the artery with one hand

- Insert the needle (25 or 26 gauge hypodermic) slowly, with the bevel up, through the skin at a 45° angle until the blood enters the syringe (sterile 1 ml to 3 ml).
- Allow 2 to 4ml of blood to enter the syringe
- Press firmly on the puncture site with sterile gauze until the bleeding stops.
- Remove all air bubbles from the sample and cap the syringe.
- Mix the sample by shaking and inverting the syringe.
- Dispose of disposable materials and sharps properly after use (sharps containers).

5.7 Material used

The blood obtained through arterial blood gases was placed in the Radiometer Copenhagen ABL 5® gas analyzer (Figure 1) to obtain the PaO2 and $PaCO_2$ variables.

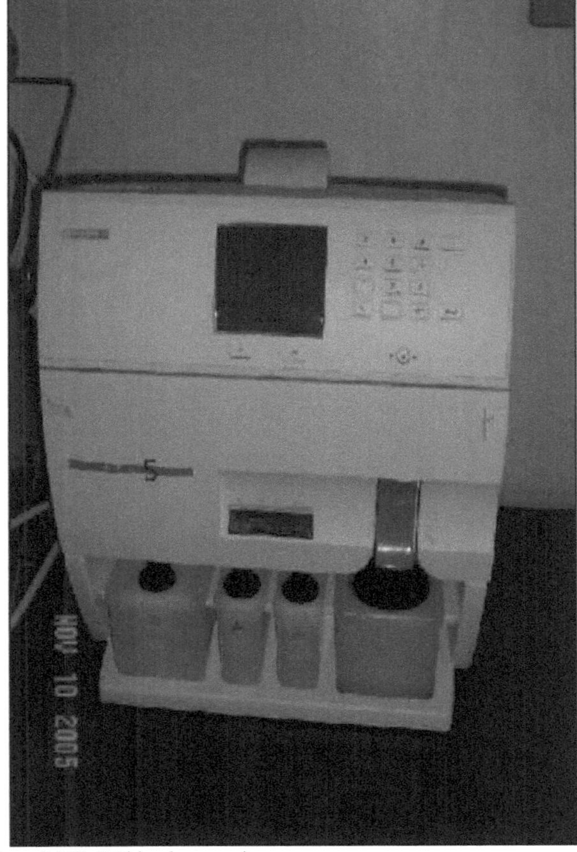

Figure 1 - Illustration of ABL 5® blood gas analyzer

5.8 Statistical Analysis

The data obtained in the survey was processed on a computer, tabulated in an Excel spreadsheet and subjected to statistical analysis using SPSS software version 10.0. All the data obtained is shown as a mean, standard deviation and in the form of graphs and tables. The significance level for the tests used was set at 95% or $p < 0.05$.

The ANOVA test was used to compare the means of the variables RR, $PaCO2$ and $PaO2$ at 24, 48 and 72 hours and the TUKEY test was used when the ANOVA test was significant to determine the difference between the intervals of the means.

The Simple Linear Correlation (appendix A) was used to analyze trends in the correlation coefficients between the variables FR x $PaCO2$, FR x $PaO2$, $PaCO2$ x $PaO2$ at 24, 48 and 72 hours.

6 RESULTS

The results obtained in our study of 55 patients, of both sexes, in the postoperative period of exploratory laparotomy due to trauma are described and presented in terms of the 1st (24 hours), 2nd (48 hours) and 3rd (72 hours) postoperative days. Table 1 shows the mean and standard deviation values for age 35.78 ± 12.59 years, anesthesia time 142.27 ± 30.95 minutes, surgery time 124.18 ± 31.43 minutes.

Table 1. Characterization of the sample in terms of lowest value, highest value, means and standard deviations in relation to age, anesthesia time and surgery time.

	Age (years)	Anesthesia time (minutes)	Surgical time (minutes)
Lowest Value	18	120	90
Highest Value	62	255	240
Average	35,78	142,27	124,18
Standard Deviation	12,59	30,95	31,43

Table 2 shows the mean and standard deviation values for RR, PaCO2 and PaO2 for the 55 patients who underwent exploratory laparotomy for trauma on the 1st, 2nd and 3rd postoperative days. The RR on day 1 was 27.49 ± 5.31 irpm, on day 2 25.35 ± 5.32 irpm and on day 3 24.15 ± 3.94 irpm. $PaCO_2$ on day 1 averaged 32.84 ± 4.49 mmHg, on day 2 33.65 ± 3.36 mmHg and on day 3 34.04 ± 3.73 mmHg. PaO2 showed a mean of 85.29 ± 18.30 mmHg on day 1, 87.53 ± 17.56 mmHg on day 2 and 89.31 ± 16.57 mmHg on day 3.

Table 2. Table showing the lowest and highest values, mean and standard deviation of respiratory rate (RR), arterial carbon dioxide pressure ($PaCO_2$) and arterial oxygen pressure (PaO_2) in the first three postoperative days.

	RR(irpm)		$PaCO_2$ (mmHg)			PaO_2 (mmHg)		
	24h	48h 72h	24h	48h	72h	24h	48h	72h

Lowest Value	20	1616	21	28	27	58	51	55
Highest Value	48	4036	42	39	42	118	122	122
Average	27,49	25,3524,15	32,84	33,65	34,04	85,29	87,53	89,31
Standard Deviation	5,31	5,323 ,94	4,49	3,36	3,73	18,30	17,56	16,57

Performing a statistical analysis to observe the variance of the means (ANOVA) in the first three postoperative days for the items RR, PaCO2 and PaO2, we observed that RR showed a p-value = 0.001787 (p < 0.05), i.e. there was a statistical difference between the means. In order to see which of the RR averages were significantly different, the Tukey test was used, which obtained a statistically significant difference for the 24-72 hour average pairs.

Applying ANOVA to $PaCO_2$, we found a value of p = 0.258079 (p > 0.05) with no significant difference between the means. For PaO_2 we found a value of p = 0.484179 (p > 0.05), likewise there was no significant difference between the means presented by the ANOVA test for the first three postoperative days.

For the O.I. we observed that on the 1st post-operative day the average was 405.44 ± 88.13, on the 2nd day the average was 414.61 ± 84.98 and on the 3rd day the average was 423.64 ± 83.17 (Table 3).

Table 3. Presentation of the lowest and highest values, means and standard deviation for the oxygenation index (OI) ratio on the first three postoperative days.

	24 hours	I.O.	
		48 hours	72 hours
Lowest Value	261,9	242,8	171,8
Highest Value	685,7	604,7	580,0
Average	405,44	414,61	423,64

Standard Deviation	88,13	84,98	83,17

In order to observe the correlation between the variables studied (RR, PaCO2 and $_{PaO2}$), a simple linear correlation was used for each postoperative day - the 1st, 2nd and 3rd days respectively - and presented in graphs.

Graph 1 shows the correlation between RR and PaCO2 on the 1st postoperative day with a value of r = - 0.42604. This r means a negative correlation with a qualitative assessment of a regular aspect between the two variables. We can see in the graph that when RR increases, $_{PaCO2}$ decreases. This correlation was statistically significant with p = 0.001182 (p < 0.01).

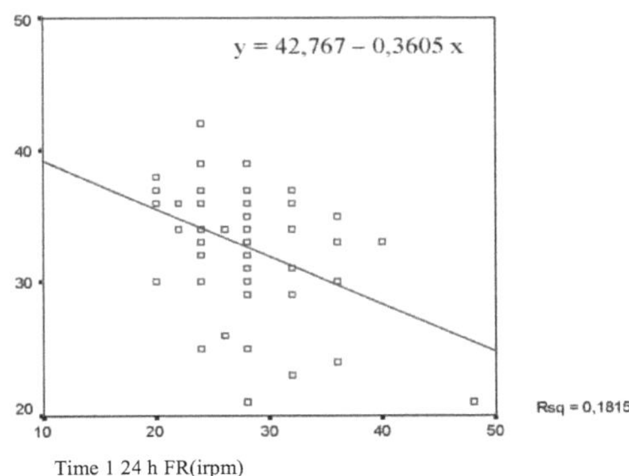

Graph 1: Graph illustrating the correlation between RR and $PaCO_2$ on the 1st postoperative day

Graph 2 shows the variation between RR and $PaCO_2$ on the 2nd postoperative day with a value of r = - 0.23857, suggesting a weak negative correlation and not being statistically significant with p = 0.079425 (p > 0.05). The straight line equation shows a negative trend, with a slight variation in RR in relation to PaCO2 on the 2nd postoperative day.

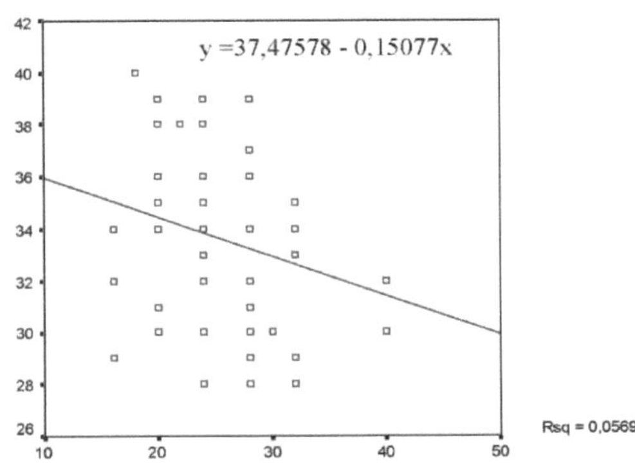

Graph 2: Graph illustrating the variation in RR x PaCO2 on the 2nd day of PO

Graph 3 shows the variation in RR and PaCO2 on the 3rd postoperative day with a value of r =-0 .02807. This r suggests a weak negative correlation and was not statistically significant with p = 0.838813 (p > 0.05). The straight line equation shows that there is no variation in PaCO2 with increasing RR.

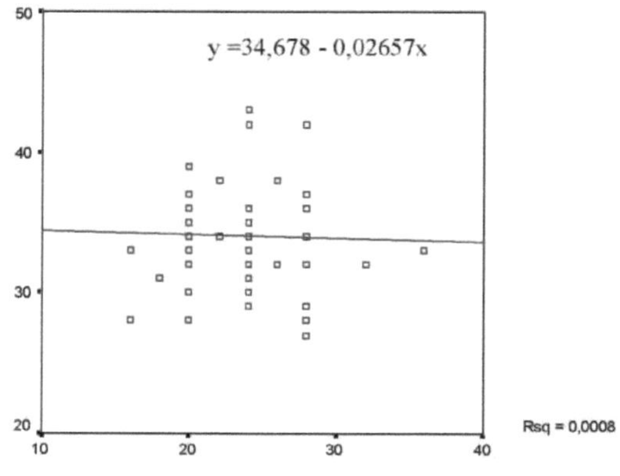

Graph 3: Graph illustrating the variation in RR x PaCO2 on the 3rd day of PO

Graph 4 shows the correlation between RR and PaO_2 on the 1st post-operative day with a value of r = - 0.28128, suggesting a weak negative correlation between these two variables and statistically significant with p = 0.037497 (p < 0.05). As RR increased, we observed a reduction in PaO_2 .

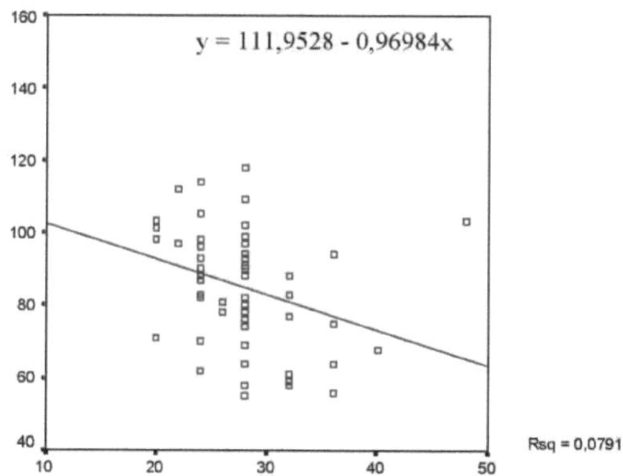

Graph 4: Graph illustrating the correlation between RR and PaO2 on the 1st PO day

Graph 5 shows the correlation of RR x PaO_2 on the 2nd postoperative day between these variables with a value of r = - 0.32166, which suggests a negative correlation with a qualitative assessment of a regular aspect and statistically significant with p = 0.016634 (p < 0.05). The straight line equation shows that as RR increases there is a reduction in PaO2 values.

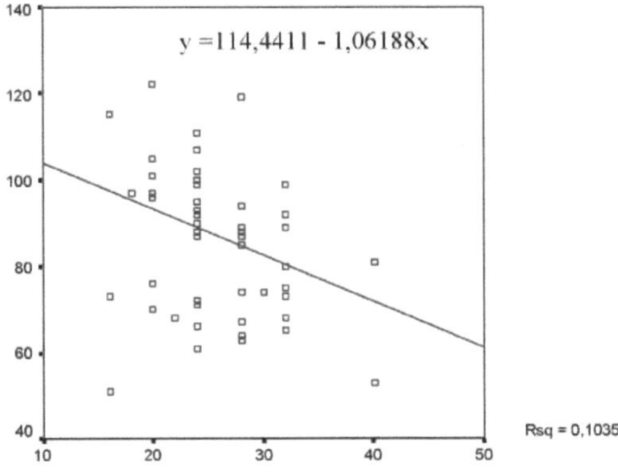

Graph 5: Graph illustrating the correlation between RR and PaO2 on the 2nd PO day

Graph 6 shows the correlation between the variables RR and PaO_2 on the 3rd post-operative day with a value of r = - 0.28597, which suggests a negative correlation and a weak and statistically significant qualitative evaluation with p = 0.034302 (p < 0.05). The straight line equation shows a tendency for PaO_2 to decrease as RR increases.

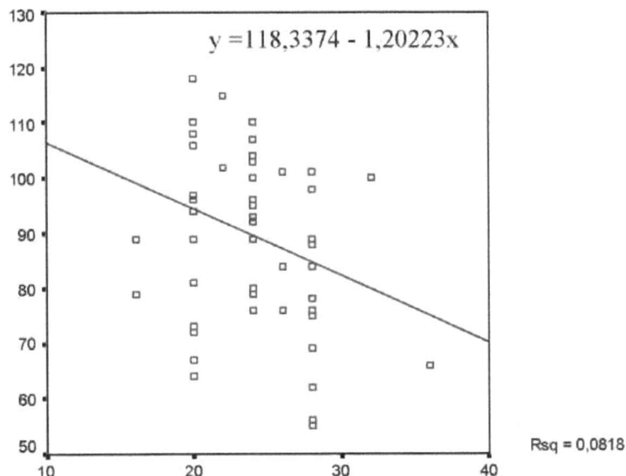

Graph 6: Graph illustrating the correlation between RR and PaO2 on the 3rd PO day

Graph 7 shows the variation between $PaCO_2$ and PaO_2 on the 1st post-operative day with a value of r = 0.023339, suggesting a weak correlation for these variables and not a statistically significant correlation with p = 0.865961 (p > 0.05). The straight line equation shows that as PaCO2 increases, PaO2 remains constant.

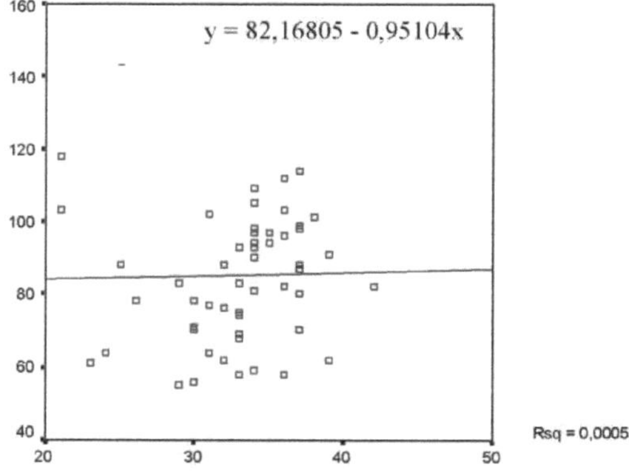

Graph 7: Graph illustrating the variation in PaCO2 x PaO2 on the 1st day of PO

Graph 8 shows the variation in PaCO2 and PaO2 on the 2nd post-operative day for these variables with a value of r = 0.2305, suggesting a weak, statistically non-significant correlation with p = 0.090446 (p > 0.05). The straight line equation shows that as PaCO2 increases there is minimal variation in PaO2 values.

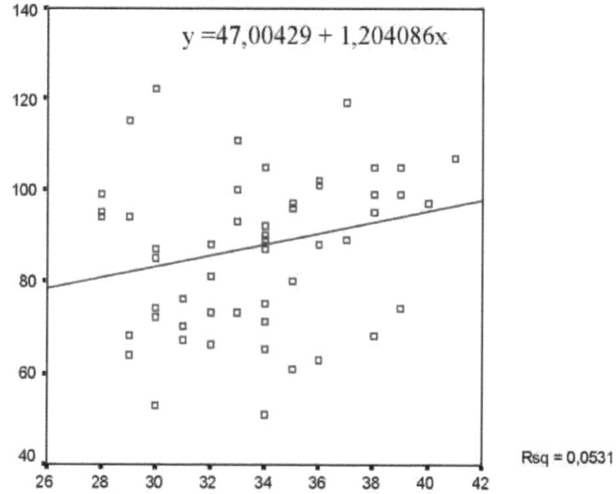

Graph 8: Graph illustrating the variation in PaCO2 x PaO2 on the 2nd day of PO

Graph 9 shows the variation between the variables $PaCO_2$ and PaO_2 on the 3rd postoperative day with a value of r = - 0.0505, which suggests a negative correlation with a weak qualitative evaluation and is not statistically significant with p = 0.714243 (p > 0.05). The graph shows the equation of the constant line with dispersion of the PaCO2 and PaO2 values.

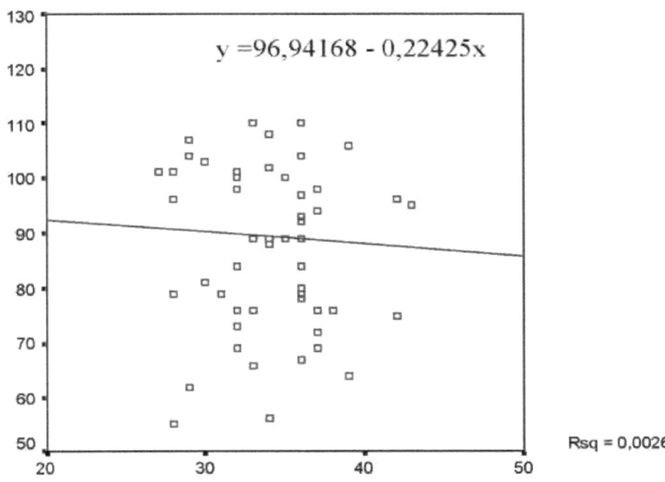

Tempo 3 72 h PaCO2(mmHg)

Graph 9: Graph showing the variation in $PaCO_2$ x PaO_2 on the 3rd day of PO

7 DISCUSSION

The appearance of post-operative pulmonary complications is very common in abdominal surgeries and can be minimized with systematic monitoring of these patients. Changes in lung mechanics due to the surgical procedure and anesthesia are factors that can contribute to postoperative complications.

Avendaña (2004) reported that abdominal trauma is more frequent in males, and that young people are the most affected. Espino et al. (2002), in their study of 359 patients admitted to the general surgery department for abdominal trauma, found that stab wounds were the leading cause of abdominal injury. In our study, there was a predominance of males and young people, with an average age of 35.78 ± 12.59 years, and the most frequent causes were firearm and stab wounds.

Although our results were not significant in terms of the variation in pulmonary ventilation and oxygenation, translated by $PaCO_2$ and PaO_2, during the follow-up period, i.e. the first three post-operative days, factors such as anesthesia time and the severity of the injury, whose average in our sample was around 142.27 ± 30.95 minutes, may have been decisive in the results obtained.

Authors such as Filardo et al. (2002), reported that surgical time of more than 210 minutes is related to a greater possibility of pulmonary complications in the postoperative period, and when associated with other risk factors, the repercussions on pulmonary function may be more evident. Guizilini et al. (2005) studied pulmonary function in patients undergoing coronary artery bypass grafting and observed a significant reduction in forced vital capacity (FVC) and forced expiratory volume in the first second (FEV_1) by the fifth postoperative day (PO), while OI showed a significant drop on the 1st PO day. In our study, OI remained within the normal range from the 1st to the 3rd postoperative day, which can be explained by the shorter surgical and anesthetic times of our patients.

Chiavegato et al. (2000) in their study, which aimed to study changes in ventilation and lung volumes and respiratory muscle strength in the postoperative period of laparoscopic cholecystectomy, observed a reduction of 26% in tidal volume, 20% in minute volume, 36% in vital capacity, 47% in inspiratory muscle strength and 39% in expiratory muscle strength on the 1st postoperative day. They also detected atelectasis in one of the patients and a return to preoperative values around the 3rd and 4th postoperative days, which is faster than in laparotomic abdominal surgeries, according to the literature. The aim of our study was not to follow the patient beyond the 3rd postoperative day.

In view of the changes in pulmonary function in the postoperative period of major surgeries, especially upper abdominal surgeries, there is a need for a consistent preoperative assessment. RAMOS et al. (2003) concluded that FEV_1, maximum oxygen consumption (VO2 max) and diffusion capacity through arterial hemogasometry are essential in the preoperative period. In our study, all the patients were referred to the operating room due to the urgent nature of the injury, which meant that strict monitoring was not possible in the preoperative and postoperative periods.

Endotracheal intubation for general anesthesia prior to the start of the surgical procedure causes alterations in the respiratory system, such as irritation of the airway, restriction of ciliary movement, especially when used for a prolonged period of time, leading to increased airway resistance and altered lung function (PRYOR & WEBBER, 2002). The ability to wean from the endotracheal tube more quickly and with less surgical time provides better performance in the postoperative period (GÓMEZ et al., 2005).

Kucukemre et al. (2005) reported that the incidence of pain in the postoperative period of abdominal surgery is significant, often requiring the administration of anesthetics in the postoperative period, with possible changes in pulmonary ventilation and oxygenation if the pain continues. They studied sixty-nine patients divided into two groups and in the postoperative morphine group they observed an improvement in parameters such as RR, arterial blood gases, pain, heart rate and blood pressure. In our study, patients were given intravenous analgesics only when necessary.

Giovanetti et al., (2004) stated that the abdominal injuries caused by the traumatic mechanism, together with the surgical procedure and the lack of mobility in bed in the postoperative period can contribute even more to the pain in this period by altering pulmonary ventilation. VIEIRA et al. (2004) confirmed that abdominal surgery contributes to respiratory muscle dysfunction, due to the pain and anesthetics used, contributing to the appearance of pulmonary complications. It is therefore believed that diaphragmatic paresis due to inhibition of the phrenic nerve as a result of manipulation of the abdominal viscera is the possible cause.

The type of anesthetic drug can also contribute to the reduction and/or alteration of some respiratory parameters. MARTINS et al., (2003) stated that the use of general anesthesia with the administration of intravenous anesthetics such as propofol and inhalation anesthetics such as isofluorane can cause changes in arterial blood gases, especially an increase in $PaCO_2$, as well as a reduction in $PaO2$ and minute volume. VASCONCELLOS et al. (2000) found no significant changes in $PaCO2$ and $PaO2$ with different concentrations of isofluorane. In our study, patients underwent general anesthesia to a similar standard using a balanced technique, intravenous anesthetics, inhalation with isofluorane and muscle relaxants, but we were unable to determine the relationship between the anesthetic used and variations in arterial gases.

Although there was no significant difference between the arterial blood gas pressures in the patients studied from the 1st to the 3rd postoperative day, we found that all the $PaCO2$ averages were below normal values at the times analyzed, and this was more pronounced on the 1st postoperative day (< 35 mmHg). The increase in RR in the PO directly interferes with pulmonary mechanics, leading to restriction of lung volume and alteration of the respiratory pattern, which may be the cause of the reduction in $PaCO2$ values. In our study, mean respiratory rates were above normal values, i.e. higher than 20 rpm from the 1st to the 3rd postoperative day, with a reduction in tachypnea as the clinical and surgical evolution progressed.

All patients were breathing at room temperature with FiO_2 at 21%, and did not require supplementary oxygen therapy. The $PaO2$ and IO averages remained within the normal range from the 1st to the 3rd postoperative day ($PaO2 > 80$ mmHg), and we also observed a recovery or increase in the $PaO2$ and $PaCO2$ values as they evolved clinically. This can be explained by the fact that the surgical time was less than 210 minutes and, as a result, arterial oxygenation was less compromised. In addition, the average age of our patients corresponds to that of young individuals, which makes their recovery in the postoperative period faster and without a history of previous lung diseases.

Oliveira Filho (2003), in his study aimed at evaluating monitoring routines and post-anesthetic discharge criteria, showed the concern of Brazilian anesthesiologists for patient safety in the immediate post-anesthetic period, reporting in decreasing order of importance the monitoring of blood pressure, heart rate, airway patency, respiratory rate, nausea and vomiting, post-operative pain and muscle strength.

Pulmonary complications can also be seen in the perioperative period due to faulty ventilation and/or intubation equipment and also in the immediate postoperative period, during post-anesthetic recovery, especially when there is no careful preoperative assessment.

In our study, as well as in others in the literature that carried out a careful preoperative assessment, we observed the need for postoperative monitoring, which should be carried out from the moment the patient leaves the operating room and PACU, detecting any alterations that could pose a risk and/or complication during the hospital stay until discharge.

Alterations in lung function such as reduced FRC and hypoxia in the postoperative period of abdominal surgery are factors that trigger the appearance of pleuropulmonary complications such as atelectasis, pneumonia and empyema. Mantovani et al. (2001) studied 110 patients with penetrating thoracoabdominal wounds who underwent exploratory laparotomy and showed that there was a greater possibility of pleuropulmonary complications, which could be explained by the fact that the lesion was located in a region where the thoracic and abdominal cavities meet, making it necessary to treat the pleura. In our study, we excluded patients who were undergoing some kind of treatment for lung damage caused by the injury, so as not to interfere with our results.

The studies reported that the rate of respiratory complications in patients undergoing exploratory laparotomy for abdominal trauma was high and that preventive measures should be taken routinely to avoid unpleasant surgical outcomes. They observed the appearance of atelectasis and pneumonia in patients undergoing the procedure, with changes in RR, PaO_2, SaO_2, VC and FVC in the first three postoperative days, which were reversed with the use of positive expiratory pressure of 08 cmH_2O twice a day for 15 minutes each. The aim of our study was not to have any kind of intervention, and no pleuropulmonary complications were detected in the first three postoperative days.

When we analyzed the influence of RR on arterial blood gases on the first three postoperative days, we found results that showed little correlation in their qualitative evaluation, which can be demonstrated by the fact that although the average RR was higher, as recommended in the literature, they were all below 30 strokes per minute, not contributing to a more obvious hypocapnia through the $PaCO_2$ values, as well as maintaining values above the normal parameter for PaO_2. However, we observed that ventilation (PaCO2) had a greater influence on the 1st postoperative day and oxygenation (PaO2) on the 1st, 2nd and 3rd postoperative days. These results can also be explained by the fact that our patients' surgery time was around 124.18 minutes, their average age was 35.78 years and certain risk factors, such as previous cardiopulmonary diseases, were excluded.

Analysis of the PaCO2 and PaO2 variables in the first three postoperative days showed no significant relationship between them, a fact that can be explained by the level of hypocapnia and the mean arterial oxygenation values without hypoxemia. Hemogasometric changes and possible trans- and post-operative complications in right intercostal thoracotomy and partial median sternotomy were compared in eighteen dogs over seven days, where no significant changes were observed in pH, blood gases and pain. In abdominal surgeries, especially laparotomic surgeries on the upper floor, the diaphragm can be damaged during surgical manipulation, which can cause changes in lung function.

Several possibilities have been raised to justify the reduction in lung volume in the postoperative period of abdominal surgery. Several factors have been mentioned in the literature that are relevant to the change in thoracoabdominal behavior during breathing, i.e. a change in the breathing pattern, making ventilation more superior, as detected on lung auscultation in practically all the patients evaluated, with a tendency to reestablishment as soon as earlier ambulation and a satisfactory clinical-surgical evolution are favored.

Comparing the various parameters studied, such as RR, PaCO2 and PaO2, RR can be considered a good measurement option for respiratory monitoring, a simple procedure to perform and easy to access for any professional accompanying the patient in the postoperative period of abdominal surgery, even serving as a determinant of the need to perform arterial blood gas. We should emphasize the importance of this marker in monitoring patient safety and anticipating possible changes in the postoperative period, and associating it with risk factors such as the severity of the injury, longer surgery time, taking greater precaution in detecting changes in blood gases such as PaCO2 and PaO2 observed by an increase in RR, with a change in breathing pattern and respiratory muscle effort.

CONCLUSIONS

Based on our results, we concluded that there was a statistical difference between the mean RR ($p<0.05$) in the first three postoperative days of exploratory laparotomy due to abdominal trauma. The significant difference between the pairs of mean RR was between 24-72 h. There was no statistical difference between the mean $PaCO_2$ and PaO2 ($p>0.05$) on the first three postoperative days. RR values were above normal (>24irpm), PaCO2 remained below the normal range (<35mmHg) and PaO2 values were above normal (>80mmHg) on the first three postoperative days. The oxygenation index remained in the normal range (>400) from the 1st to the 3rd postoperative day. We observed a statistical correlation between RR and $PaCO_2$ on the 1st postoperative day ($p<0.05$) and between RR and PaO_2 on the 1st, 2nd and 3rd postoperative days ($p<0.05$). There was no statistical correlation between PaCO2 and PaO2 on the first three postoperative days ($p>0.05$). The use of RR as an easily accessible and low-cost parameter makes postoperative patient monitoring a safe and fundamentally important way of assessing clinical and surgical progress and detecting possible changes in pulmonary mechanics.

REFERENCES

AIRES, M. M. **Fisiología**. 4th edition. Rio de Janeiro: Guanabara Koogan, 2012.

AMERICAN ASSOCIATION FOR RESPIRATORY CARE. Clinical practice guideline: Sampling for arterial blood gas analysis. **Respir. Care.** v.37, 1992.

AVENDAÑA, J. Carballo. Complications from exploratory laparotomy for blunt trauma of the abdomen at the Dr. Roberto Calderón Gutiérrez School Hospital, January 1999 - December 2003. **Managua.** s.n. 2004.

BARRETO NETO, P. F. et al. Colorectal trauma: a retrospective study. **Rev. Bras. Colo-proctol.** v.22, n.3, 2002.

BARROS, J.A. **Preoperative pulmonary evaluation in candidates for elective general surgery**. [Master's thesis - Escola Paulista de Medicina, 2000].

BICKENBACH, K. A., KARANICOLAS, P. J., AMMORI, J. B., JAYARAMAN, S., WINTER, J. M., FIELDS, R. C., BRENNAN, M. F. "Up and down or side to side? A systematic review and meta-analysis examining the impact of incision on outcomes after abdominal surgery". **The American Journal of Surgery**, v. 206, n. 3, p. 400-409, 2013.

BRIENNON, X., LERMITE, E., MEUNIER, K., DESBOIS, E., HAMY, A., & ARNAUD, J. P. "Surgical treatment of large incisional hernias by intraperitoneal insertion of Parietex® composite mesh with an associated aponeurotic graft (280 cases)". **Journal of visceral surgery**, v. 148, n. 1, p. 54-58, 2011.

BROOKS-BRUNN, J.A. Predictors of postoperative pulmonary complications following abdominal surgery. **Chest**, v. 111, 1997.

CALLEGARI-JAQUES, S. M. **Biostatística: principios e aplicares**. Sao Paulo: Artmed, 2004.

CALLINS, V.J. **Princípios de anestesiologia**. 2.ed. Rio de Janeiro: Guanabara-Koogan, 1978.

CAMHI, S.; ENRIGHT, P.L. How to assess pulmonary function in older persons. **J. Resp. Diseases**, v.21, n.6, 2000.

CARDIM, E. **Pre- and post-operative respiratory assessment in patients undergoing elective upper abdominal surgery for digestive disorders**. [Thesis presented to the Federal University of Sao Paulo - EPM], 1991.

CARVALHO, Carlos R.R. **Ventilado mecánica**. Sao Paulo: Atheneu, 2000.

CELLI, B.R. Preoperative respiratory careof the patient undergoing upper abdominal surgery. **Clin Chest Med**, v. 14, 1993.

CHIAVEGATO, L.D. et al. Respiratory functional changes in laparoscopic cholecystectomy. **J. Pneumol.**, v.26, n.2. 2000.

CHRISTENSEN, E.F. et al. Postoperative pulmonary complications and lung function in high-risk patients: a comparison of three physiotherapy regimens after upper abdominal surgery in general anesthesia. **Acta Anaesthesiol. Scand.** v.35.1991.

CUSCHIERI, R.J. et al. Postoperative pain and pulmonary complications: comparison of three analgesic regimens. **Br. J. Surg.**, v.72. 1985.

DE ARRIBA-ARNAU, A., DALMAU, A., SALVAT-PUJOL, N., SORIA, V., BOCOS, J., MENCHÓN, JM, URRETAVIZCAYA, M. "Induction of hypocapnia and hyperoxia using a hyperventilation protocol in electroconvulsive therapy." **Revista de Psiquiatría y Salud Mental** , v. 10, n. 1, p. 21-27, 2017.

DESPREZ, K., MCNEIL, J. B., WANG, C., BASTARACHE, J. A., SHAVER, C. M., WARE, L. B. "Oxygenation Saturation Index Predicts Clinical Outcomes in ARDS." **Chest**, v. 152, n. 6, p. 1151-1158, 2017.

DIOGO FILHO, A.; ROCHA, Savassi P.R. **Pre-operative**. In: ROCHA, Savassi P.R. Abdome agudo. Rio de Janeiro: Guanabara-Koogan, 1982. In: ROCHA, P.R.S. et al. **Abdome agudo:** diagnóstico e tratamento. 2.ed. Rio de Janeiro: Medsi, 1993.

DUREVIL, B. et al. Effects of upper or lawer abdominal surgery on diaphragmatic function. **Br.J.Anaesth.** v.59, 1987.

EMMERICH, Joao C. **Respiratory monitoring and fundamentals.** Rio de Janeiro: Livraria e Editora Revinter Ltda, 2011.

EPSTEIN, S.K. et al. Predicting complications after pulmonary resection. Preoperative exercise testing vs a multifactorial cardiopulmonary risk index. **Chest**, v. 104.1993.

FARESIN, S.M. et al. Risk factors for pulmonary complications in the postoperative period of upper abdominal surgery. Sao Paulo. **J. Pneumol**, v.22. 1996.

FARROE, S.C. et al. Epidemiology in anesthesia II: Factors affecting mortality in hospital. **Br.J.Anesthesiol.**, v. 54. 1982.

FERNANDES, C. R. & NETO, P. P. R. The respiratory system and the elderly: anesthetic implications. **Rev. Bras. Anestesiol.** v.52, n.4. 2002.

FERRAZ, E.M. **Wound infection in digestive tract surgery.** Recife: Federal University of Pernambuco, 1990

FILARDO, F. A.; FARESIN, S. M.; FERNANDEZ, A. L. G. Validity of a prognostic index for the occurrence of pulmonary complications in the postoperative period of upper abdominal surgery. **Rev. Assoc. Méd. Bras.** v.48, n.3. 2002.

FILARDO, F.A. **Validation of a prognostic index for pulmonary complications in the postoperative period of elective upper abdominal surgery.** Sao Paulo, 1998 [Master's thesis - Federal University of Sao Paulo].

FORD, G.T. et al. Diaphragm function after upper abdominal surgery in humans. **Am. Rev. Respir. Dis.**, v. 127.1983.

FREEMAN, L.J.; NIXON, P.G.F. Chest pain and the hyperventilation syndrome: some etiological considerations. **Postgraduate Medical Journal.** v.61. 1985.

GALVÄO, L. **Cirurgia do aparelho digestivo** Rio de Janeiro: Guanabara-Koogan, 1978.

GARDNER, W.N.; BASS, C. Hyperventilation in clinical practice. **British Journal of Hospital Medicine.** v.41,n. 1. 1989.

GIOVANETTI, E.A.; BOUERI, C.A.; BRAGA, K.F. Comparative study of lung volumes and oxygenation after the use of Respiron and Voldyne in the postoperative period of upper abdominal surgery. **Reabilitar.** v.6. n.25, 2004.

GOFFI, F. S. **Surgical technique:** anatomical and pathophysiological bases and surgical techniques. 5.ed. São Paulo: Atheneu, 2010.

GOLDMAN, L.; BRAUNWALD, E. General anesthesia and noncardiac surgery in patients with heart disease. In: **Braunwald E.** Heart disease. 4th .ed. Philadelphia: W.B. Saunders Company, 1992.

GUIZILINI, S.; GOMES, W. J.; FARESIN, S. M.; BOLZAN, D. W.; ALVES, F. A.; CATANI, R.; BUFFOLO, E. Evaluation of pulmonary function in patients undergoing coronary artery bypass grafting with and without cardiopulmonary bypass. **Braz. J. Cardiovasc. Surg.** v.20, n.3. 2005.

GUNDEL, O., GUNDERSEN, S. K., DAHL, R. M., JORGENSEN, L. N., RASMUSSEN, L. S., WETTERSLEV, J., MEYHOFF, C. S. "Timing of surgical site infection and pulmonary complications after laparotomy." **International Journal of Surgery**, v. 52, p. 56-60, 2018.

GUYTON, A.C.; HALL, J.E. **Treatise on Medical Physiology.** 13ª ed. Rio de Janeiro, Elsevier Ed., 2017.

HAAHR-RAUNKJ^R, C., MEYHOFF, C. S., S0RENSEN, H. B. D., OLSEN, R. M., AASVANG, E. K. " Technological aided assessment of the acutely ill patient-The case of postoperative complications". **European journal of internal medicine**, v. 45, p. 41-45, 2017.

HERNÁNDEZ-GRANADOS, P., LÓPEZ-CANO, M., MORALES-CONDE, S., MUYSOMS, F., GARCÍA-ALAMINO,J., & PEREIRA-RODRÍGUEZ, J. A. "Incisional Hernia Prevention and Use of Mesh. A Narrative Review". **Cirugía**

Española (English Edition), 2018.
HERRING, P. J., RIPPIN, B. "Anaesthesia for abdominal vascular surgery".
Anaesthesia & Intensive Care Medicine, v. 14, n. 5, p. 200-203, 2013.
HINES, R.L. The anesthetic management of the failing heart. **Sem.Anesth**, v. 9. 1990.
HOPPER, K. "Respiratory Acid-Base Disorders in the Critical Care Unit." **Veterinary Clinics of North America: Small Animal Practice,** v. 47, n. 2, p.351-357, 2017.
HOROVITZ, J.H. et al. Pulmonary response to major injury. **Arch Surg.**, v. 108. 1974.
JACKSON, C.V. Preoperative pulmonary evaluation. **Arch. Intern. Med.,** v.48. 1988.
JAITLY, V. K., KUMAR, C. M. "Continuous spinal anesthesia for laparotomy."
Current Anaesthesia and Critical Care, v. 20, n. 2, p. 60-64, 2009.
JEFFREY, CC. Et al. A prospective evaluation of cardiac risk index. **Anesthesiol.** v.58. 1983.
JONES, R., BERRY, R. "Mechanisms of hypoxaemia and the interpretation of arterial blood gases." **Surgery-Oxford International Edition,** v. 33, n. 10, p. 461-466, 2015.
KUCUKEMRE, F.; KUNT, N; KAYGUSUZ, K.; KILICCIOGLU, F.; GURELIK, B.; CETIN, A. Remifentanil compared with morphine for postoperative patient-controlled analgesia after major abdominal surgery: a randomized controlled trial**. Eur. J. Anaesthesiol.** v.22, n.5. 2005.
LARKIN, B.G.; ZIMMANCK, R.J. "Interpreting arterial blood gases successfully."
AORN journal, v. 102, n. 4, p. 343-357, 2015.
LAWRENCE, V.A. et al. Risk of pulmonary complications after elective abdominal surgery. **Chest**, v. 110. 1996.
LECKY, J.H.; OMINSKY, A.J. Postoperative respiratory management. **Chest**, v. 62 (Suppl), 1972.
LEQUEUX, B., UZAN, C., REHMAN, M. B. "Does resting heart rate measured by the physician reflect the patient's true resting heart rate? White-coat heart rate. " **Indian Heart Journal**, 2017.
LÓPEZ, M.; MEDEIROS, J.L. **Semiologia médica:** as bases do diagnóstico clínico. 5.ed. Rio de Janeiro: Livraria e Editora Revinter Ltda, 2004.
MACFIELD, G.; BURKE,D. Parasthesia and tetany induced by voluntary hyperventilation. **Brain**, v. 114. 1991.
MAGALHÁES, H.P. **Surgical technique and experimental surgery**. Sao Paulo: Sarvier, 1996.
MANGANO, D.T. Perioperative cardiac morbidity. **Anesthesiol.**, v. 72. 1990.
MANICA J. et al. **Anesthesiology**: principles and techniques. 3.ed. Porto Alegre: Artes Médicas, 2004.
MANTOVANI, M.; FONTELLES, M; AJUB, J. R.; PINTO, F. S. Incidence of pleuropulmonary complications in thoracoabdominal injuries. **J. Bras. Med.** v.81, n.2. 2001.
MARTINS, S. E. C.; NUNES, N.; REZENDE, M. L. de ; SANTOS, P. S. P. dos. Effects of desfluorane, sevofluorane and isofluorane on respiratory and hemogasometric variables in dogs. **Braz. J. Vet. Res. Anim. Sci.** v.40, n.3. 2003.
MEDEIROS, R.A. **Pulmonary complications and postoperative mortality in patients undergoing elective general surgery**. Sao Paulo, 1997 [Master's thesis - Federal University of Sao Paulo].
MELENDEZ, J.A.; CARLON, V.A. Cardiopulmonary risk index does not predict complications after thoracic surgery. **Chest**, 1998.
MOHAMMED, H. M., ABDELATIEF, D. A. "Easy blood gas analysis: Implications for nursing." **Egyptian Journal of Chest Diseases and Tuberculosis**, v. 65, n. 1, p. 369-376, 2016.
NAIK, B. I., COLQUHOUN, D. A., SHIELDS, I. A., DAVENPORT, R. E., DURIEUX, M. E., BLANK, R. S. "Value of the oxygenation index during 1-lung

ventilation for predicting respiratory complications after thoracic surgery." **Journal of critical care**, v. 37, p. 80-84, 2017.

NAMPOOTHIRI, M.; BOYARS, M.C. Why the dry cough and recent dyspnea? **J. Resp Diseases**, v.21, n.4, 2000.

NORMANDO, V.; COSTA, D. DEL-TETTO, C.; NORMANDO, R. Utilization of positive pressure with face mask in the prevention of respiratory complications of abdominal trauma. **Rev. Para. Med.** v.15, n. 4. 2001.

OLIVEIRA FILHO, G. R. de. Post-anesthetic care routines of Brazilian anesthesiologists. **Rev. Bras. Anestesiol.** v.53, n.4. 2003.

OLIVEIRAA, L.T., ESSUA, F. F., MESQUITAA, G. H. A., JARDIMA, Y.J., IUAMOTOA, L. R., SUGUITAA, F.Y., MARTINES, D.R., NII, F., WAISBERG, D.R., MEYER, A., ANDRAUS, W., D'ALBUQUERQUE, L.A.C. "Component separation of abdominal wall with intraoperative botulinum A presents satisfactory outcomes in large incisional hernias: a case report." **International journal of surgery case reports**, v. 41, p. 99-104, 2017.

OLIVER, C.M., WALKER, E., GIANNARIS, S., GROCOTT, M. P. W., MOONESINGHE, S. R. "Risk assessment tools validated for patients undergoing emergency laparotomy: a systematic review". **BJA Advance Access Published,** 2013.

OPPERSMA, E., DOORDUIN, J., VAN DER HOEVEN, J. G., VELTINK, P. H., VAN HEES, H. W. H., & HEUNKS, L. M. A. "The effect of metabolic alkalosis on the ventilatory response in healthy subjects." **Respiratory physiology & neurobiology**, v.249, p. 47-53, 2018.

PAISANI, D.M. et al. Volumes, lung capacities and respiratory muscle strength after gastroplasty. **J. Brás. Pneumol**, v.31 n.2. 2005.

PEDERSEN, T. et al. A prospective study of risk factors and cardiopulmonary complications associated with anaesthesia and surgery risk indicators of cardiopulmonary morbidity. **Acta Anaesthesiol. Scand.**, v. 34. 1990.

PEDERSEN, T.; RINGSTED, C. Postoperative pulmonary complications following surgery: influence of general and regional anesthesia. **Acta Anaesthesiol. Scand.** v.34. 1990.

PEREIRA, E.D.B. et al. Risk factors for pulmonary complications in the postoperative period of upper abdominal surgery. **J. Pneumol.**, v. 22, n.1. 1996.

PEREIRA, E.D.B. et al. Prospective assessment of the risk of postoperative pulmonary complications in patients submitted to upper abdominal surgery. **Sao Paulo Med. J.**, v. 117, n.4, 1999.

PINTO, M. P. S. F.; KOZLOWSKY, G.; STOPIGLIA, A. J.; FREITAS, R. R.; FANTONI, D. T.; SIMOES, E. A.; BINOKI, D. H. Comparative study between intercostal thoracotomy, partial and total median sternotomy in healthy dogs (*canis familiaris*): Clinical and hemogasometric evaluation. **Acta Cir. Bras.** v.15, n.4. 2000.

PIRAS, C.A. Gasometria arteriale na relação tempo entre recolha e realização do exame. **Rev. Bras. Terapia Intensiva.** v.14, n.3, 2002.

PRYOR, J. A.; WEBBER, B. A. **Physiotherapy for respiratory and cardiac problems.** 2.ed. Rio de Janeiro: Guanabara Koogan, 2002.

QURESHI, S. M., MUSTAFA, R. "Measurement of respiratory function: gas exchange and its clinical applications." **Anaesthesia & Intensive Care Medicine**, v. 19, n. 2, p. 65-71, 2018.

RAMOS, G.; RAMOS FILHO, J.; PEREIRA, E.; JUNQUEIRA, M.; ASSIS, C. H. C. Preoperative evaluation of the pneumopath. **Rev. Bras. Anestesiol**. v. 53, n. 1. 2003.

RAO, T.L.K. et al. Reinfarction following anesthesia in patients with myocordial infarction. **Anesthesiol**, v.59, 1983.

REDONDO GÓMEZ, Z. A.; CORDOVÍ DE ARMAS, L.; VALLONGO MENÉNDEZ, M. B.; REDONDO GÓMEZ, R. Laryngeal mask vs. endotracheal tube in long-term surgical interventions. Clinical trial. **Rev. Argent. Anestesiol.** v.63, n.3. 2005.

RIBEIRO-SILVA, A.; SILVA, G.A. Intrapulmonary gas exchange under room air breathing in hypercapnic patients. **Rev. Assoc. Med. Bras.** v.50, n.1.2004.

RIESER, T. M. "Arterial and venous blood gas analyses." **Topics in companion animal medicine**, v. 28, n. 3, p. 86-90, 2013.

ROCHA, N.A. **Smoking as a risk factor for pulmonary complications and mortality in the postoperative period of elective upper abdominal surgery**. Sao Paulo, 1998 [Master's thesis - Federal University of Sao Paulo].

ROCHA, P.R.S. et al. **Acute abdomen:** diagnosis and treatment. 2.ed. Rio de Janeiro: Medsi, 1993. RONDON ESPINO, J. A.; AGUILAR DOMINGUEZ, L. C.; ROJAS BARTHELEMY, I; GARCIA HERNÁNDEZ, I.; OJEDA OJEDA, M. J. Traumas abdominales. Experiencia en un Servicio de Cirugía General, 1986 a 1993. **Rev. Cuba Cir.** v.41, n.2. 2002.

ROYSTER, R.L. Causes and consequences of arrhythmias. In: BENUMOF, J.L.; SAIDMAN, L.J. Anesthesia and perioperative complication. St Louis, **Mosby Year Book,** 1992.

SAAD, I.A.B.; ZAMBOM, L. Clinical variables of preoperative risk. **Rev.Assoc.Med.Bras.,** v.47, n.2. 2001.

SAHNI, A. S., GONZALEZ, H., TULAIMAT, A. "Effect of arterial puncture on ventilation." **Heart & Lung: The Journal of Acute and Critical Care**, v. 46, n. 3, p. 149-152, 2017.

SANTOS JÚNIOR, J. C. M. dos. Risk factors associated with surgical complications in operations involving resection and anastomosis of the large intestine without mechanical preparation: study of the incidence of infection and anastomotic dehiscence. **Rev. Bras. Colo-proctol.** v.25, n.2. 2005.

SCANLAN, C. L. WILKINS, R. L.; STOLLER, J. K. **Egan's Fundamentals of Respiratory Therapy.** Sao Paulo: Manole, 2000.

TANG, H., LIU, D., QI, H. F., LIANG, Z. P., ZHANG, X. Z., JIANG, D. P., ZHANG, L. Y. "Effect of retension sutures on abdominal pressure after abdominal surgery." **Chinese Journal of Traumatology,** v. 21, n. 1, p. 20-26, 2018.

TAZIMA, M.F.GS., VICENTE, Y.A.M.V.A., MORIYA, T. "Laparotomy". **Medicina (Ribeirao Preto. Online),** v. 44, n. 1, p. 33-38, 2011.

TIPPING, R., BERRY, R., NESBITT, I. "Mechanisms of hypoxaemia and the interpretation of arterial blood gases." **Surgery-Oxford International Edition**, v. 33, n. 10, p. 461-466, 2015.

VASCONCELLOS, C. H. C.; ÁRSICO FILHO, F.; GOMEZ SEGURA, I. A.; NASCIMENTO, P. R. L.; MONTEIRO, R. V. Utilization of isofiorane in capuchin monkeys. **Braz. J. Vet. Res. Anim. Sci.**v.37, n.1. 2000.

VIEIRA, G. B.; BREGAGNOL, R. K.; SANTOS, A. C. B.; PAIVA, D. N. Evaluation of the effectiveness of transcutaneous electrical nerve stimulation on pain intensity, lung volumes and respiratory muscle strength in the postoperative period of abdominal surgery: a case study. **Rev. Bras. Fisioter.** v.8. n.2. 2004.

WARNER, D.O. et al. Airway obstruction and perioperative complications in smokers undergoing abdominal surgery. **Anesthesiol.,** v. 90. 1999.

WAY, L. W. **Surgery:** diagnosis and treatment. 14.ed. Rio de Janeiro: Guanabara-Koogan, 2017.

WHITE, P.F. **Tratado de anestesia venosa**. 1. ed. Porto Alegre: Artmed, 2003.

WILLIAMS, R S., KOZAN, P., SAMOCHA-BONET, D. "The role of dietary acid load and mild metabolic acidosis in insulin resistance in humans." **Biochimie**, v. 124, p. 171-177, 2016.

WONG, D.H. et al. Factors associated with postoperative pulmonary complications in patients with severe chronic obstructive pulmonary disease. **Anesthesiol. Analg.,** v. 80.

1995.
WONG, S. S. C., IRWIN, M. G. "Anaesthesia and minimally invasive surgery." **Anaesthesia & Intensive Care Medicine,** v. 19, n. 1, p. 11-15, 2018.
YEAGER, M.P. et al. Epidural anesthesia and analgesia in high-risk surgical patients. **Anesthesiol.** V. 66. 1987.
ZINGG, T., BHATTACHARYA, B., MAERZ, L. L. "Metabolic acidosis and the role of unmeasured anions in critical illness and injury." **Journal of Surgical Research,** v. 224, p. 5-17, 2018.

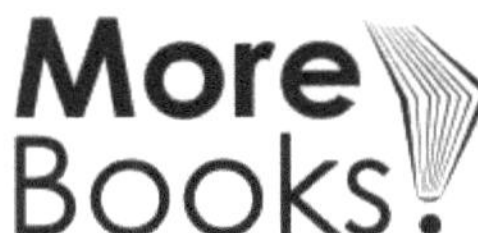

More
Books!

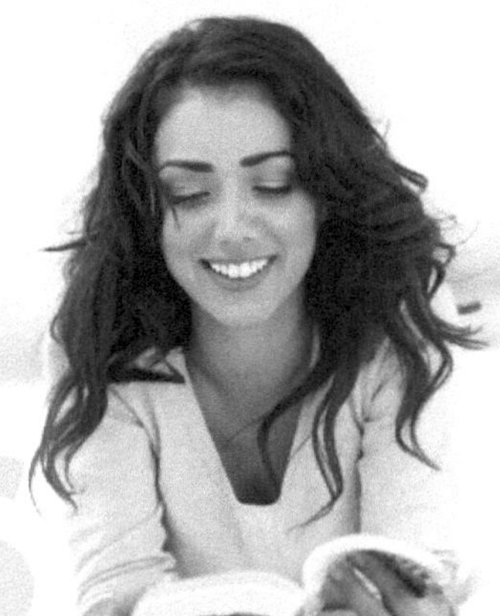

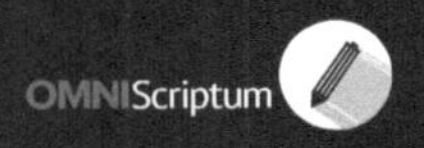

info@omniscriptum.com
www.omniscriptum.com
OMNIScriptum

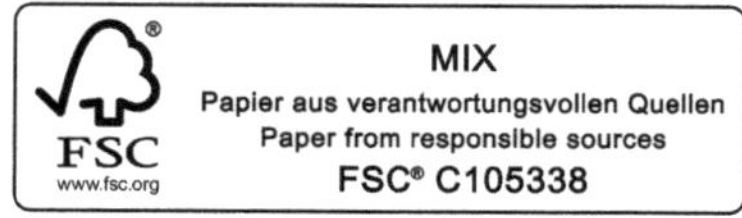